W9-ABQ-309

ENCYCLOPEDIA OF HUMAN NUTRITION

SECOND EDITION

ENCYCLOPEDIA OF HUMAN NUTRITION

SECOND EDITION

Editor-in-Chief
BENJAMIN CABALLERO

Editors
LINDSAY ALLEN
ANDREW PRENTICE

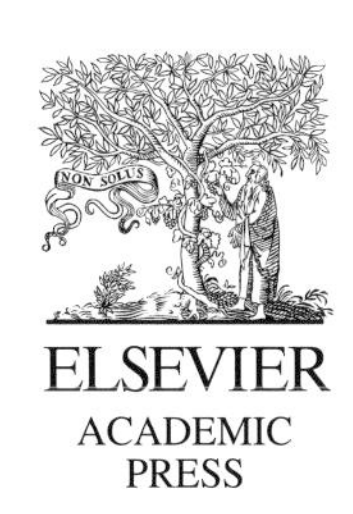

ELSEVIER
ACADEMIC
PRESS

Amsterdam Boston Heidelberg London New York Oxford
Paris San Diego San Francisco Singapore Sydney Tokyo

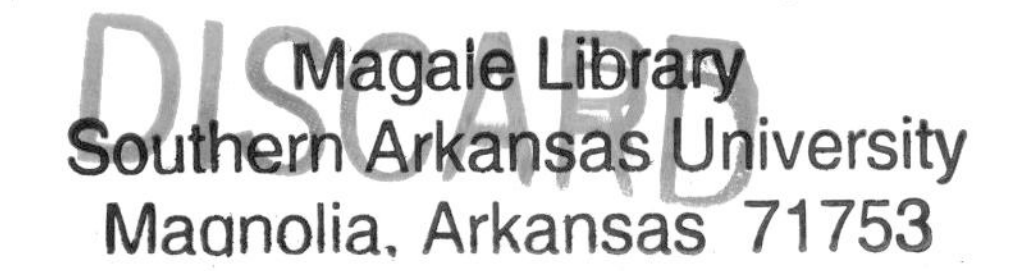

Elsevier Ltd., The Boulevard, Langford Lane, Kidlington, Oxford, OX5 1GB, UK

Second edition 2005

Library of Congress Control Number: 2004113614

A catalogue record for this book is available from the British Library

ISBN 0-12-150110-8 (set)

This book is printed on acid-free paper
Printed and bound in Spain

EDITORIAL ADVISORY BOARD

FOREWORD

Why an encyclopedia? The original Greek word means 'the circle of arts and sciences essential for a liberal education', and such a book was intended to embrace all knowledge. That was the aim of the famous Encyclopedie produced by Diderot and d'Alembert in the middle of the 18th century, which contributed so much to what has been called the Enlightenment. It is recorded that after all the authors had corrected the proofs of their contributions, the printer secretly cut out whatever he thought might give offence to the king, mutilated most of the best articles and burnt the manuscripts! Later, and less controversially, the word 'encyclopedia' came to be used for an exhaustive repertory of information on some particular department of knowledge. It is in this class that the present work falls.

In recent years the scope of Human Nutrition as a scientific discipline has expanded enormously. I used to think of it as an applied subject, relying on the basic sciences of physiology and biochemistry in much the same way that engineering relies on physics. That traditional relationship remains and is fundamental, but the field is now much wider. At one end of the spectrum epidemiological studies and the techniques on which they depend have played a major part in establishing the relationships between diet, nutritional status and health, and there is greater recognition of the importance of social factors. At the other end of the spectrum we are becoming increasingly aware of the genetic determinants of ways in which the body handles food and is able to resist adverse influences of the environment. Nutritionists are thus beginning to explore the mechanisms by which nutrients influence the expression of genes in the knowledge that nutrients are among the most powerful of all influences on gene expression. This has brought nutrition to the centre of the new 'post-genome' challenge of understanding the effects on human health of gene-environment interactions.

In parallel with this widening of the subject there has been an increase in opportunities for training and research in nutrition, with new departments and new courses being developed in universities, medical schools and schools of public health, along with a greater involvement of schoolchildren and their teachers. Public interest in nutrition is intense and needs to be guided by sound science. Governments are realizing more and more the role that nutrition plays in the prevention of disease and the maintenance of good health, and the need to develop a nutrition policy that is integrated with policies for food production.

The first edition of the Encyclopaedia of Human Nutrition established it as one of the major reference works in our discipline. The second edition has been completely revised to take account of new knowledge in our rapidly advancing field. This new edition is as comprehensive as the present state of knowledge allows, but is not overly technical and is well supplied with suggestions for further reading. All the articles have been carefully reviewed and although some of the subjects are controversial and sensitive, the publishers have not exerted the kind of political censorship that so infuriated Diderot.

John Waterlow.

J.C. Waterlow
Emeritus Professor of Human Nutrition
London School of Hygiene and Tropical Medicine
February 2005

INTRODUCTION

The science of human nutrition and its applications to health promotion continue to gain momentum. In the relatively short time since the release of the first edition of this Encyclopedia, a few landmark discoveries have had a dramatic multiplying effect over nutrition science: the mapping of the human genome, the links between molecular bioenergetics and lifespan, the influence of nutrients on viral mutation, to name a few.

But perhaps the strongest evidence of the importance of nutrition for human health comes from the fact that almost 60% of the diseases that kill humans are related to diet and lifestyle (including smoking and physical activity). These are all modifiable risk factors. As individuals and organizations intensify their efforts to reduce disease risks, the need for multidisciplinary work becomes more apparent. Today, an effective research or program team is likely to include several professionals from fields other than nutrition. For both nutrition and non-nutrition scientists, keeping up to date on the concepts and interrelationships between nutrient needs, dietary intake and health outcomes is essential. The new edition of the Encyclopedia of Human Nutrition hopes to address these needs. While rigorously scientific and up to date, EHN provides concise and easily understandable summaries on a wide variety of topics. The nutrition scientist will find that the Encyclopedia is an effective tool to "fill the void" of information in areas beyond his/her field of expertise. Professionals from other fields will appreciate the ease of alphabetical listing of topics, and the presentation of information in a rigorous but concise way, with generous aid from graphs and diagrams.

For a work that involved more than 340 authors requires, coordination and attention to detail is critical. The editors were fortunate to have the support of an excellent team from Elsevier's Major Reference Works division. Sara Gorman and Paula O'Connell initiated the project, and Tracey Mills and Samuel Coleman saw it to its successful completion.

We trust that this Encyclopedia will be a useful addition to the knowledge base of professionals involved in research, patient care, and health promotion around the globe.

Benjamin Caballero, Lindsay Allen and Andrew Prentice
Editors
April 2005

GUIDE TO USE OF THE ENCYCLOPEDIA

Structure of the Encyclopedia

The material in the Encyclopedia is arranged as a series of entries in alphabetical order. Most entries consist of several articles that deal with various aspects of a topic and are arranged in a logical sequence within an entry. Some entries comprise a single article.

To help you realize the full potential of the material in the Encyclopedia we have provided three features to help you find the topic of your choice: a Contents List, Cross-References and an Index.

1. Contents List

Your first point of reference will probably be the contents list. The complete contents lists, which appears at the front of each volume will provide you with both the volume number and the page number of the entry. On the opening page of an entry a contents list is provided so that the full details of the articles within the entry are immediately available.

Alternatively you may choose to browse through a volume using the alphabetical order of the entries as your guide. To assist you in identifying your location within the Encyclopedia a running headline indicates the current entry and the current article within that entry.

You will find 'dummy entries' where obvious synonyms exist for entries or where we have grouped together related topics. Dummy entries appear in both the contents lists and the body of the text.

Example

If you were attempting to locate material on food intake measurement via the contents list:

FOOD INTAKE *see* DIETARY INTAKE MEASUREMENT: Methodology; Validation. DIETARY SURVEYS. MEAL SIZE AND FREQUENCY

The dummy entry directs you to the Methodology article, in The Dietary Intake Measurement entry. At the appropriate location in the contents list, the page numbers for articles under Dietary Intake Measurement are given.

If you were trying to locate the material by browsing through the text and you looked up Food intake then the following information would be provided in the dummy entry:

Food Intake *see* **Dietary Intake Measurement**: Methodology; Validation. **Dietary Surveys. Meal Size and Frequency**

Alternatively, if you were looking up Dietary Intake Measurement the following information would be provided:

DIETARY INTAKE MEASUREMENT

Contents

Methodology

Validation

2. Cross-References

All of the articles in the Encyclopedia have been extensively cross-referenced.

The cross-references, which appear at the end of an article, serve three different functions. For example, at the end of the ADOLESCENTS/Nutritional Problems article, cross-references are used:

i. To indicate if a topic is discussed in greater detail elsewhere.

> *See also*: **Adolescents**: Nutritional Requirements of Adolescents. **Anemia**: Iron-Deficiency Anemia. **Calcium**: Physiology. **Eating Disorders**: Anorexia Nervosa; Bulimia Nervosa; Binge Eating. **Folic Acid**: Physiology, Dietary Sources, and Requirements. **Iron**: Physiology, Dietary Sources, and Requirements. **Obesity**: Definition, Aetiology, and Assessment. **Osteoporosis**: Nutritional Factors. **Zinc**: Physiology.

ii. To draw the reader's attention to parallel discussions in other articles.

> *See also*: **Adolescents**: Nutritional Requirements of Adolescents. **Anemia**: Iron-Deficiency Anemia. **Calcium**: Physiology. **Eating Disorders**: Anorexia Nervosa; Bulimia Nervosa; Binge Eating. **Folic Acid**: Physiology, Dietary Sources, and Requirements. **Iron**: Physiology, Dietary Sources, and Requirements. **Obesity**: Definition, Aetiology, and Assessment. **Osteoporosis**: Nutritional Factors **Zinc**: Physiology.

iii. To indicate material that broadens the discussion.

> *See also*: **Adolescents**: Nutritional Requirements of Adolescents. **Anemia**: Iron-Deficiency Anemia. **Calcium**: Physiology. **Eating Disorders**: Anorexia Nervosa; Bulimia Nervosa; Binge Eating. **Follic Acid**: Physiology, Dietary Sources, and Requirements. **Iron**: Physiology, Dietary Sources, and Requirements. **Obesity**: Definition, Aetiology, and Assessment. **Osteoporosis**: Nutritional Factors. **Zinc**: Physiology.

3. Index

The index will provide you with the page number where the material is located, and the index entries differentiate between material that is a whole article, is part of an article or is data presented in a figure or table. Detailed notes are provided on the opening page of the index.

4. Contributors

A full list of contributors appears at the beginning of each volume.